I Was So Bipolar

A Look Back at 2007

By Terri Kovalcik

Edited By Amy Lignor

Terri Kovalcik
I WAS SO BIPOLAR

Terri Kovalcik
I WAS SO BIPOLAR

Printed in Canada

ISBN:- 13: 978 1497499812

ISBN 10: 149749981X

All the characters in this book are fictitious, and any resemblance to persons living or dead is purely coincidental.

Terri Kovalcik
I WAS SO BIPOLAR

This book is dedicated to the world, so they can better understand the bipolar community.

Acknowledgements

I could not have written this book without being inspired by Employment Counsellor, Deanna Kubas. I could not have drawn on my experiences without my parents, ex-husband, son, adopted family, cherished friends, the unmedicated, and the people I have worked for and beside. Even though a majority of the experiences have been hurtful, the whole situation has made me a stronger person. Perhaps a little too hard, but what can you expect from a bipolar? Answer: Nothing lesss than twice your 'maxed-out' feelings.

A very special thank you to Amy Lignor who has now passed on, who brought such hope, self-confidence, and love to my sister heart.

Terri Kovalcik
I WAS SO BIPOLAR

Do you have friends or family that suffer from depression? If so, do you wonder why they are they way they are? If you're looking for quick facts, what symptoms to look for, and explanations for the expressive behaviours of your loved one, you may have found a stimulating book that provides examples and thoughts concerning what it's like to be bipolar...

Table of Contents

Terri Kovalcik
I WAS SO BIPOLAR

Introduction

Exception
By Terri Kovalcik

defining an existence
among society
standing
only one
an individual set forth into this world

Being a rapid cycler, my overly- abundant thoughts come at maximum speed. Multiple subjects are constantly being played inside my brain, like an endless montage where problem solving is as natural as every breath I take. My double-edged sword has taken me down the path of writing, creating a book that will give the reader a better understanding of what it's like to be classified as a "Bipolar disordered" person living in today's society. This is the day and age where it sounds like everyone and their dog is bipolar, yet no one understands what this disability can do... and destroy.

I am not a doctor, or a scientist, or a counsellor; I am a single individual on life's journey who's experiencing things that I wouldn't wish on my worst enemy. I have an ability to look at my life and make fun of it. After all humor helps. Some of my own favourite quotes are: "Life without laughter is life a puddle without water," and "Life is like a stage; there are actors that play parts in our lives that help establish us, allow us to grow as individuals."

I am an authority on my bipolar disordered life. From the first traumatic event to almost dying to find a goal that helped experience joy; learn that I could be too intense at times, yet not enough in relationships; to allowing me to accomplish a complete '180'- taking my previous life experience and beginning the Full Treatment Program.

My work life is not the one I wanted. I never entered a job with the hopes of being fired or having to leave it because of this recurring disability that has overtaken me. I dreamed of having a job that would last at least five years but, with the world around me, the reality is that it's not going to happen in the 'normal' 9-to-5 workforce.

I'd like to think I'm not a typical Bipolar. I enjoy reading books that help me grow spiritually as an individual and realize why things in my life have happened on this journey of self discovery and acceptance. You can't change the past, as we all know, you can only learn from it and try your best not to repeat your errors as the world revolves around us and time moves forward. It is a given that each generation- each person- has their own evolution.

My life changed a great deal when a relationship came to an end because of repeated exposure to anxieties that simply don't goo away; the problems were intensified because I was under-medicated. My condition worsened and I knew I had to change, because if I didn't, I would continue to make the same mistakes. This is when I read *The Road Less Traveled, Touched With Fire*, and the incredibly popular *Men are From Mars, Women are From Venus.* Each one combined to enhance my ability to 'call it like it is', despite the look of shock on the faces of the people around me when I admitted the bipolar disorder. More often than not when you voice a conclusion it leaves an unsettling feeling of remorse, even though it's the truth. I can't help but tell the truth because lying to yourself only works for so long; blaming everyone else for the problems that have occurred simply stops working. The old saying, "Life is what you make it"" is definitely true.

I have cell phone, dial-up internet, a disability, social, and employment anxieties, and an eating disorder that still overtakes me at times because it feels like the world is not quite ready for me. The question is: Will you be ready for a bipolar disordered person when you've finished reading this book? I hope so. That person needs emotional support in order to take a disability and turn it into an asset that works for them and not against them. But only time will tell if the following words will give you strength and courage to be the understanding friend another person needs.

What It's Not

Judgement
By Terri Kovalcik

I lie here in my shallow grave
I hear voices
I hear what they say
they think I am dead
but I am very much alive
judgement will be their undoing
as their graves
will be shallower than mine

Bipolar is not curable, and it definitely is not a virus. It is not a physical, or a mental capacity defect. It is not obvious or easily diagnosed. You are not born with this alienating disability that affects approximately one in five people with mood disorders, and women are more likely to have it.

As much as one cannot say it is a virus, it may feel like a close relative. Unlike society, this disability doesn't discriminate against age, sex, religion, sexual or political preference.

I WAS SO BIPOLAR

There are various ways, or possible causes of how one can experience an episode. It's believed to be in the DNA of our ancestors, just a small speck that sits with its other emotional "pals", like depression and happiness. As we all know, every person has stress. When the biochemical that's released within that body when work-related stress, relationship turmoil, or financial fear occurs, we begin to feel a slight annoyance but, as long as the stress lingers that feeling increases ten-fold, creating anxieties that are lifelong and will never go away no matter how many prescriptions your doctor, psychologist, or psychiatrist tell you to take.

Scientists say that there is no single thing that causes bipolar, it stems from many factors acting together. There have been studies of identical twins to see if both have bipolar disorder but, what they have found out is that that one will have it, while that the other is more likely to develop the illness then, say, another sibling.

Scientists have been looking for other genes that creates the illness but are having a difficult time discovering them.

Knowing that no bipolar disordered person experiences the exact same thing – every encounter, relationship, life's crappy moments, and greatest joys- aren't the same. My level of excitement is different than someone else, and even more different when un-medicated. These levels show the world what a pendulum of emotions human beings are capable of experiencing. It is said that we bipolar disordered people create many faces of extreme feelings. When I was under-medicated, I went from extremely happy to sad and crying in less than a minute. That's when I called my family doctor and accepted the fact that I needed a mood stabilizer. You see, at one time, I was in control of my medication. It must've driven my doctor nuts but, then again, all under-medicated bipolar disordered people are severely stubborn. My dosage was increased, but then I had to sit down and visit with the 'pill prescribing psychiatrist' who didn't realize that she overdosed me with Sequel. She had upped my family doctor's prescription by three, creating pain in the back of my head. I will never again let anyone else other than myself prescribe pills, seeing as that the three different kinds of chemicals that she 'experiment with' made me incredibly ill.

This is one of the reasons why I didn't want to take medication, because it could me very ill, or act differently. I was put on anti-depressants to ease the second traumatic event in my life- giving birth- but at the time I was worried that my husband wouldn't pay for them, and I didn't want to start taking a pill if I would not be able to afford it the next month. It only took my eleven years to acknowledge and accept the fact I would be taking medication for the rest of my life. After all, it took ten years just to get diagnosed.

Hit Me with Your Best Shot

Situation
By Terri Kovalcik

a placement
in life
destituted to be

fate
or a
mockery

thoughts
questions

speaking out
stopping
listening
changing

Among the pile of research about bipolar, I came across something that I still find rather amusing. It needs to be said that there are individuals out there who seem to think that God has bipolar and He's an ultra-rapid cycler. These people ask that we understand and have patience with Him. In my opinion, if there was such a thing, why does God have a personality disorder? Is not God the all-powerful, all-knowing omnipresence that created Man in His image? If He did then every Tom, Did, Harry, Sally, or Sue should have bipolar disorder, not just the five percent of the worlds' population. It is amazing how the brain works and it perceives events. I haven't imagine blaming God for swift acts like tornadoes, extreme weather conditions, or when someone who has been seriously ill recovers only to have die, or have a permanent disability. Two million Americans, eighteen years or older in any given year, has bipolar disorder. And symptoms can occur during childhood, as well as develop late in life.

How do we catch this disability? The onset begins with a traumatic physical or emotional event with a combination of several factors influencing that individual's life. The bipolar DNA is passed down from generation to generation. These people have mild to severe depression and, then a traumatic event happens releasing the chemical imbalance. It can take years before this disability is diagnosed because most people with bipolar don't want to admit what it is, how it affects their lives, and cannot accept taking chemical prescriptions for the rest of their lives.

I look back on my life and first traumatic event took place when I was nine years old. It was summertime; the strawberries were ready to be picked. My brother and I lived in a 'negative attention' world, and every year my dad would pay us to pick Saskatoon's, wild strawberries etc. I was in the wild strawberry patch picking berries for my dad when my brother told me that was his patch. Like normal children we argued, and I picked up a small rock and threw it at the front tire of his bike. My brother responded by picking up a bigger rock and, when my back was turned, threw it at my head. Blood began gushing from my head as I fell to my knees crying. Are you wondering what my older sibling did? He ran back to the house and into his room, crying all the way. I was rushed to the hospital; my dad never drove so fast in his life. While I was being stitched up it felt as though I was looking down on my body, and ever since then if I lay a certain way it feels like I'm having an out-of-body experience.

Terri Kovalcik
I WAS SO BIPOLAR

My condition escalated at the age of nineteen. I wed too young, because my parents wanted me married off so they wouldn't have to worry about me anymore. Married at nineteen and had my first child in September of the next year. We were young, my husband and I. We grew up completely different but had one thread that was similar- low self- esteem. He was three years older than me and if it wasn't for the fact that my mother set the wedding date, I wouldn't be where I am at today.

Being pregnant was not a pleasant experience but, what can you expect from a person who grew up in a verbally abusive house? After giving birth to my son, I, like most women, got the 'baby blues' but, mine was far worse. He was born early due to stress, and we were in the hospital for a week because his liver was fully developed, which added to my depression.

Now I reflect on the past and cry, because I wish that I never had bipolar disorder, or any type of depression. I wish that I didn't have such horrible mood swings so that my life experiences couldn't been celebratory instead of painful. But no matter how many times I look back on my life, the past cannot be changed.

The Un-Medicated

Oblivion
By Terri Kovalcik

**a swinging chord
entertaining
amusement
and
wonder**

What can you say about the un-medicated other than the fact that there are far too many people out there who aren't doing the *Full Treatment Program?* By not taking the medication you could almost compare them to a cyclone of chaos. Their condition worsens every single time a traumatic even occurs. Frustrating moments in life are continually happening, creating anxieties that become more and more apparent to the point of absurdity to 'normal' people. They don't listen to the solutions; they only want to whine about the problems. They are bull-headed with extreme mood swings, and their highs and lows are frequent. They seem to have this special power that's like a metal detector going off when it finds something with a metallic element buried in the ground, except that their bell starts ringing loudly when they find someone else with a similar affliction to their own. There should be a huge warning label on these people, and I should've had one as well, because if either or both parties are un-medicated, both anxiety levels with be the same... and that's not healthy. For example: depressed, anxious, frustrated- they are simply creating a path of destruction for both of them. They can be the 'Drama Queens' for the 'pity pot'; they are dangerous with credit and most end up in bankruptcy. They do things that aren't right and, more often than not, they are substance abusers.

The tag of 'substance abuser' is a perception and most don't consider that illegal substance to be harmful. In my research, I've found that most are cocaine addicts. I completely disagree, based on my own self. There may be individuals out there who start off with the mild stuff like marijuana only to then move on to experience elevated 'emotions' that are produced by crack, cocaine, crystal meth, acid, ecstasy, and other chemically produced illegal substances. I can see it being very easy for some to dive deeply into the substance abuse, not wanting to admit what the real problem is, and that their substance of choice worsens their condition unless regulated by the individual. Because of my disability and core values, I'll never turn to chemical drugs because I've seen what it does to 'normal' people. Once they start taking those harsher drugs they have to continue for the rest of their lives- it's not a choice anymore.

I have come across some people, that even with my disability, I see as complete opposites of me and it's horrifying. I met this one person who was off their meds because they believed the prescription wasn't' helping. Of course, they didn't' feel right because, without the meds, they had powerful mood swings, and made mountains out of molehills just to get attention. They carried on and on about how horrible their life has been for three hours as they retold their life story to me -an endless tale of unfinished events that made them look weak and in desperate need of help.

I am always for the underdog and, let me tell you, it has kicked me in the butt a great many times. I tried to help- which was dumb of me- but I believe in the good of all people. This person was the Drama Queen winner of all the un-medicated I have ever encountered. With this person I tried to be the problem solver, I always am. I suggested solutions to their problems. Well, let me tell you how that went. Oh, my word! It was the biggest mistake of my life! The 'pity pot' came into play and this person lied to me to get sympathy. I suggested getting away from the anxieties that were stemming from their living conditions, which resulted in me being asked to look after a dog... and I did. What a mistake that; I was now responsible for a dog that was only supposed to stay a couple of days which turned into almost two weeks. The excuses that were given to me to 'smooth' over the fact that this person should've been back weeks ago, was that they had discs in their neck disintegrating which meant that they weren't supposed to drive anywhere for a while. The next excuse was that they vehicle was in an accident, funny thing is that the van didn't have a dent in it. When this person finally showed up at my house, they angered me with their 'feel sorry for me' garbage, including the fact that they had massive financial problems. At first, I started out with suggestions to help solve the issue, but every choice was turned down. Inc conclusion, I choices to free myself from the situation. I didn't want this person in my life anymore and emailed a letter stating that fact. All part of life's evolution.

The Full Treatment Program

Unfounded
By Terri Kovalcik

I am lost unfound
beneath the sands of time
waiting to be discovered
to take new shape
I wait for thee

waiting, wondering, hoping
sleeping beneath the layers
unfound
I wait for thee

time travel onwards
but only darkness falls upon my eyes

If you know a bipolar who is following the recommended plan of:

- Taking proper dosages of medication consistently
- Seeing the family doctor monthly
- Visiting an Interior Health counsellor every 2 weeks
- See a Psychiatrist every 6 weeks
  Then I suggest you call **Ripley's Believe It or Not**
  Just kidding

Proper prescription dosage is mandatory and needs to be carefully determined by weight, height, age, sex, and severity of the condition. Otherwise, the patient may become ill if over medicated. If under-medicated, the condition will worsen faster than without any medication at all. This is something I should know. It has happened to me.

Again, I am no doctor. Therefore, I have no background or education to talk about the different kinds of prescriptions that are available. What works for me may not work for someone else, and side effects that I've experience may not occur for someone else.

What I can talk about is that, just because you are on medication doesn't mean that an episode won't occur. One example is financial anxieties; not having enough money to pay your bills each month. Decisions have to be made and, in this scenario, and this is where the episode can stat and will continue to escalate if you let these worries consume you. I have found a medication yet that nullifies any anxieties that I have.

In the case of due diligence, I must be honest about getting on the *Full Treatment Program* as soon as possible, by telling you hat I have not found a family doctor that I like. Or if I have found one, they are closed practice but will take you as a walk-in.

In my little town of 100 Mile House, all the medical clinics take walk-ins. This is great for me because of my cell phone anxiety which has overlapped to land-line phones. I realize that having a regular doctor is important, but I'm not ready to seek one out immediately. I had a wonderful family doctor who amazed me by quickly providing answers to the problems I was having at the time. As for the pain in the back of my head, the problem was that "there are no nerves in my brain and that was just a headache". Well, 'haa haa haaa' on that one. Turns out that the pain I was experiencing was caused from being overdosed. So, as you can understand, I am not too inclined to seek out another doctor consider this past episode.

My very first doctor didn't stick around much. I don't hold it against him. I was simply un-medicated, and under-medicated during his care. In fact, as soon as he got in the room he wanted to run away. I never opened-up, and 'fought' against taking medication but I was an unhappy person for quite some time.

In order to maintain a sense of stability I see a counsellor every two weeks. So many things happen to bipolars when it comes to mood swings, perceptions, and daily events that happen during a two-week period that counsellor is necessary. Especially being a rapid cycler who's on a mission to get better and get over the anxieties I have.

Although I stated seeing the Psychiatrist in July of 2007 it wasn't working until 2013 When I met Dr. Ronald Chale out of the Kamloops Royal Inland Hospital. My meds are correct, and I'm functioning in society better than ever.

Our appointments are only thirty minutes long where I present a chart on my mood swings, sleep patters, life events that happen over each two-week period. I have to say, "Get Real" when it comes to keeping charges consistently up to date. I haven't been able to do it, but I have tracked any productivity of writing by making smiley faces on the calendar for the past three years. That must count for something.

I started a journal for different areas in my life, but it's been about a month since I wrote anything down in it. This would be a problem for bipolars if they have small attention spans but true intentions to keep tables on themselves.

Taking medications that are supposed to stabilize moods is important, because there's nothing like being an 'emotional pendulum' going from ecstatic crying to rage within moments of haring some event that affects you on a psychological level.

I've read about bipolar common traits. It says that we have strained interpersonal relationships. Mine are with my parents, brother, and sister in-law, - well to be honest- all family members. So, the uncomfortable silences and misspoken words are accurate when it comes to strained relationships.

Counseling can't express enough; the importance of having someone to help you through the hurt and see patterns is a necessity. According to the research it says that a bipolar should have cognitive behavioural therapy because it's supposed to help change inappropriate or negative thought patterns and behaviours associated with the illness. Psychoeducation is supposed to teach me what my illness and treatment are all about, along with how to recognize symptoms so that they don't get out of hand.

Part of the *Full Treatment Program* talks about family. If most bipolars are the same there's no sense of family, therefore, having Family Therapy sessions may seem almost pointless even though it's supposed to help deal with that this disability has done to the 'family unit'. (Good luck with that). There is even therapy to help improve interpersonal relationships, regularize daily routines, and sleep patterns which are supposed to minimize manic episodes. This therapy is called Interpersonal and Social Rhythm Therapy.

If the episodes are bad and the mood swings are huge, one can ask for an ECT, which is Electroconvulsive Therapy. I never had one so I wouldn't know what it's like other than to joke about it and say, if you and your doctor don't agree, ask to be tasered by a friendly police officer. (I'm only joking, but it is a funny mental picture.)

Taking herbal supplements like St. John's Wort hasn't been studied long enough or well enough yet, so I wouldn't take it because it's not covered by medical.

See that? There are all kinds of issues when it comes to the *Full Treatment Program* so be prepared.

Bipolar: Which Degree Are You?

Perception
By Terri Kovalcik

Calmly, swiftly reach into the depths
pulling something unknownst to me

Hearing life and its' evil thoughts
shudder and recognize that
it's only me

Fear creeps upon me
The ugly blackness rears its forsaken head
its' face twisting insecurity into my heart

POOF

When I began my mission to write this book, I went into the project thinking that only a couple of kinds of bipolar exist. Well, as it turns out, there are many classifications of bipolar disorder and Mood Disorders. ***The Diagnostic and Statistical Manual of Mental Disorders*** (DSM-IV) offers a list under the heading *Dysthmic Disorder and Major Depressive Disorder* that reads: bipolar disorder categories are Bipolar 1, Bipolar 2, and Cyclolthymic Disorder. There are mood disorders caused by general medical conditions, as all as substance induced mood disorders.

The International Statistical Classification of Diseases and Related Health Problems (Tenth Revision) provides a more in depth look at the severity of related disorders with bipolar categorized as being part of the world of "affective disorders". This is the listing of ICD-10 Mood Disorders along with the severities.

Manic Episode:

- Hypomania
- Mania without psychotic symptoms
- Mania with psychotic symptoms
- Other mania episodes
- Manic episode, unspecified

Bipolar Affective Disorder:

- Current episode hypomania
- Manic without psychotic symptoms
- Manic with psychotic symptoms
- Mild or moderate depression
- Severe depression with psychotic symptoms
- Episode is mixed
- In remission
- Other bipolar affective disorders
- Bipolar affective disorder unspecified

Depressive Episode:

- Mild depressive episode
- Moderate depressive episode
- Severe depressive episode without psychotic symptoms
- Severe depressive episode with psychotic episode
- Other depressive episodes

- Depressive episode, unspecified

Persistent Mood (Affective) Disorders:

- Cyclothymia
- Dysthymia
- Other persistent mood (affective) disorder
- Unspecified

Recurrent Depressive Disorder:

- Current episode is mild
- Episode is moderate
- Severe without psychotic symptoms
- Severe with psychotic symptoms
- In remission
- Other recurrent depressive disorders
- Unspecified

Other Mood (Affective) Disorders Unspecified Mood (Affective) Disorders:

There is a classification system which distinguishes the sux subtypes of manic depression that is referred to "Young and Klerman Subtypes"

Bipolar 1:   Mania and Major Depression

Bipolar 2:   Hypomania and Major Depression

Bipolar 3:   Cyclothymia

Bipolar 4:   Antidepressant induced Hypomania

Bipolar 5: Major Depression with a family history of
Bipolar Disorder
Bipolar 6: Unipolar Mania

Repeated Exposure

101
By Terri Kovalcik

**Basic
Rudimentary
Natural
Obvious
The way it is**

So far, I haven't read any information about what the factors or definition of repeated exposure is, or what it can do if not corrected. I can only tell you that when something occurs to you repeatedly for more than one month, in my book it constitutes as repeated exposure.

This repeated exposure can and will disrupt your life patterns just likes it's disrupting mine at this very moment while I am writing this book. My episode right now is being caused by a dog who continually stares at as they are eating. The dog almost runs to the kitchen like his tail is on fire when it hears the fridge door open. Each time that door is open- there's the dog. You pull out the frying pan drawer- there's the dog. You open a cupboard.... Well, you get the point. There isn't even peace in the bathroom, and if you put boot or shoes on, the dog follows you everywhere just waiting for you to head outside. It lies in front of the couch so close that you can't put your feet down on the floor. It wants to sit with you on the couch and will continue to stare at you until you give in. When it's bedtime, there he is again. Oh, and my personal favorite, is that this medium-sized dog is allowed its very own personal furniture- the love seat where it sleeps and puts on quite the show.

This is what I call repeated exposure. I've been trying to deal with this issue for over six months. The problem likes in the difference of opinion on what a dog should eat and what the dog should or shouldn't rest on. The biggest problem is that I'm not used to having a pet that continually stares at me and follows me everywhere. I have an eating disorder so, perhaps, the dog continually staring at me because it's a social issue, - I don't like eating in front of other people without offering them food as well.

Being under-medicated and then over-medicated and trying to stabilize on the current dosages of medication didn't help this relationship. In the beginning it was all good- the dog was placed outside or shut in the bedroom during the course of the meal. Unfortunately, at 'snacky' times and with repeated exposure the anxieties came. I now have anxieties about eating, because if I go to the kitchen before, I put the dog behind a door, the dog is there staring at me which makes it impossible to eat. It got to the point of insanity for me, and when my boyfriend was at work, I would just put the dog outside. My eating disorder soon disappeared and I wasn't angry with the dog anymore. I even gained some weight which is a good thing because I usually don't eat until two or three o'clock in the afternoon. Things have changed again, and my eating disorder is acting up again. I'm getting angry with the dog, and I have no compassion for it, especially when it doesn't use its brain and take cover when it's raining outside. Instead, the canine Drama Queen sits on the back deck in the farthest corner and stays there until I let it back in. I have watched. I have listened to it bark at me, telling me to let it in and I refuse, because I will not have some animal dictate to me their needs.

Yes, to most I seem mean, but to the world is just a big "sissy" when it comes to this kind of stuff. But the world is not a sissy when it comes countries are at war fighting over issues that they should think about before heading straight into bloodshed. That's a dream world, isn't it? So, not being a sissy about a dog who has attained facial expressions that make it look it's sitting in a cage located in hell or looks like I'm going to beat on it as it remains constantly in my way, is not going to break me. Won't know what I'm trying to do to overcome these feeling of rage from being stared at all the time? It's funny, it must be. Otherwise, I'd be moving out of this residence so fast because of the feelings I'm having towards the dog. I got my adopted nephews to create a variety of pumpkin faces and I cut each one out and taped them all over the house. I didn't feel I had enough, so I made twenty-three, or so more. So now whenever I go, I have unique faces staring back at me making me smile. This definitely helps me and the dog.

Another case of repeated exposure would be my phone anxieties. Every time my ell phone rang I would either lose the call before I would able to get a proper signal, or try to make a call but couldn't because I was in a two bar analog/no cell phone service area. I would try to send text messages only to have them fail sixty percent of the time. The cell phone service that was inside my residence would bounce from two bars analog/one bar digital to no service whatsoever at leave four times in one minute. Can you imagine how frustrating that could be? I hate my phone. I was beyond angry every time I answered it, and most of the time never answered it because by the time I got to the place where I could get service, I would lose the call. Can you hear me now? Nope. Never?

I went through this for seven months, and the last three were brutal. I couldn't afford to have a cell and a land line, and I still have problems even nine months (still in 2023) later. It took two weeks to call my writing support group and remind them of a meeting the next day. As with everything…. Some days are way better than others.

Anxieties

The Ever Present Light
By Terri Kovalcik

raindrops falling
swiftly, pouring
dripping, sopping
daintily like tiny ballerinas
twirling swiftly down to the
pugent smelling earth

golden rays light up the horizon
have to touch
must feel
I would love to be the golden rays
showing such care and deep concern
loving gently, here and there

must try to feel the golden rays when
the raindrops are falling,
dripping making their presence known to all

This is another topic that I haven't found too much information about when doing my extensive research, except- of course- for the -Wikipedia- version.

What causes anxieties? Repeated exposure is what I say. My anxiety about being the 'new employee' at an established place of business falls under the repeated exposure category. It is social. In essence, he anxiety of everyone wanting to get to know you at first, then when they don't like you anymore, they have you fired. The other part is fear, because I don't want to get involved in any new interpersonal relationships I end up looking like the anti-social cow.

Another area of this fear steams from my disability and how passionate I am in the customer service industry. The belief of wanting to treat people the way I want to be treated – with respect- is already 'set' in my brain. Every person that walks through the door is the reason why I have job, period. As you can see it's quite the dilemma. I want to work but I don't want people attaching themselves to me. I want to sell products but can't because of fear concerning other employees' insecurities. My perception is that they will begin to look like at their productivity and feel like they're going to lose their job because their job performance does not and will never equal mine. Do you see the double-edged sword? Can't excel because no one understands or accepts who you are, and the fact that what you have is something you cannot change.

My eating anxieties are the same thing; the dog staring at me and the fear that the dog will stare at me while I'm trying to eat something also stems from the fear. Being bipolar offers a great deal of "issues" that must be overcome.

How It Works

How Do The Fall?
By Terri Kovalcik

How do the fall
to the left
to the right
or do you sit in the middle

quest or questions
to seek answers
only to find them
in ourselves

come on
let's get off of the fence
seek the questions

The best way to explain how bipolar works is to tell you what the symptoms of various disorders are. The most important thing that has to be considered is that mood swings don't just happen; they come from a build up of emotions, various perceptions and environmental factors.

Signs that would make you eligible for the Bipolar 2 label:

- One or more major depressive episodes
- At least one hypomanic episode

36

I WAS SO BIPOLAR

There has never been a manic or mixed episode; Another disorder is not responsible for symptoms and

- Systems cause distress or impair functioning

Typical Signs of Depression

- Decreased energy
- Weight loss or gain
- Hopelessness
- Grumpy
- Chronic pains that are not caused from a physical activity previous to onset of pain
- Thoughts of death (this is a symptom) (If you had what bipolars have you'd wish death too as it destroys relationships, job opportunities, self employment opportunities, and the fact that you never stop feeling alone)

Emotions a person would display if in a hypomania episode

- Grandiosity (everyone seems to think I suffer from this on a regular basis)
- Decreased need for sleep (sometimes, but only if I forget to take my nighttime meds. When this happens your brain over fires thus making it, so you don't get any sleep)
- Pressured speech (oh for sure. I talk super fast, especially when I'm excited about my new project, and when I'm trying to explain something under stressful conditions)

- Racing thought (my thoughts don't particularly race; they are like a steady stream of various thoughts entering and exiting my conscious mind at one time)
- Spending sprees (guilty as charged but getting better)
- To do thing without properly thinking things through (that is based on how fast a brain works)
- Excess energy (mine come from my antidepressants)
- Distractible (Always. I have a short attention span on a regular basis. I want to know what's going on around me, but other times when I'm focused like I am now, I will not stop unless I absolutely have to stop writing because I gotten to the point where I'm ignoring everyone else in my life.)

The difference between Bipolar 1 and Bipolar 2 is that number 2's has hypomanic episodes but not manic one, which means the severity of the episodes don't quite impair a person's daily function or cause the need for hospitalization. That is a perception again, because the bipolar may not see anything wrong with their actions even though the other person in the room might believe that person is in desperate need of hospitalization. If you have hallucinations or paranoia, it's supposed to mean that you have Bipolar 1. Manic depression alters your moods and thoughts regular even with medication. When depressed, one can begin to imagine that the relationship they're in is in detrimental. They believe that their partner doesn't care because of small things, like only making enough food for them. In reality, all of these little things add up to this destructive thought. Mood swings can range from being enrage to grumpy and crying. They are very much like a pendulum unless medication is taken and closely monitored.

I WAS SO BIPOLAR

The manic episode is when the bipolar is happy and has three or more symptoms for most of the day, for one week, or even longer.

The great thing about being in a hypomania state is the fact that one can multitask. This is quite normal because I more productive when my medications are right and with self regulated substance use. I can accomplish at least six tasks, including writing if I'm on a regular routing that includes being by myself for an eight-hour day, and the dog is outside.

When I go through a depression phase I can feel utterly worthless. I can feel like I have made several terrible mistakes that could be constituted as a crime, and I don't feel like I'm ever going to be published, or self employed because of bipolar disorder and the other psychological and environmental factors that influence my life. Included in the environmental factors are the financial anxieties due to lack of money and the inability to have the employment I want because of who I am. Imagine going from thinking that self employment is attainable because I created my business plan (and it's a great one that will be successful) to suddenly believing it's not – that I will never be a success no matter what. When I think about how m corporation will be run and hiring managers to run various departments it all works.

But then my anxiety starts up because the world doesn't know what I have unless I tell them and when I tell they don't understand. I'm a Donald Trump fan, so when he says, "You have to have believe in what you are selling" Just times the effect that has on me and multiply it by three when I'm un-medicated. Seventy-five percent of the time I went into the local schools to the test the market of Junior Hunters at Large series, I walked out of the office with a check in my hand. That is the power of belief when used to its fullest potential.

The intensity of an unmedicated bipolar disordered person is unbelievable. The depth of feelings is too much for anyone, including the bipolar. And the poser of the 'love' emotion can only be explained like this: you will never have a normal relation with a bipolar.

A Long Ways Yet To Go

Rising Above the Noise
by Terri Kovalcik

Come clear of the fog
walk into the sun
form a distance everything looks small
but as one walks
into the picture
to recreate with creativity
whatever it may be
hold it in its entirety
see teh world for what it is
either to change it
or live amongst it

Remember I said life is what you make it? It's true. You have a choice to be sad or happy. If we sit in the 'pity pot' and talk about everything that's going wrong in your life then, yes you will be depressed- just like having an episode. You're the one who is in charge of the severity of the feelings that you're experiencing. The cyclone of chaos for the un-medicated is that, as soon as an incident occurs, they are on the phone calling friends for sympathy, and they tell the tale several times which makes the episode escalate.

Terri Kovalcik
I WAS SO BIPOLAR

I've heard of the un-medicate on the phone calling everyone that they know and, and if that person wasn't home, they left and in0depth message about events that had just occurred. Everyone does this, but the absurdity of the bipolar mind when it's escalating is way out there. For example: in baseball, hitting a grand slam is awesome and rare, with the feeling of excitement and adrenaline pumping through the veins. Now that that feeling and reverse it, having the same exact 'high' but a feeling of distress. Crazy huh?

The world isn't cheering you on when you jut had in your perception a grand slam of a bad event and, quite honestly, nobody wants to hear it. I am calling it how it is because we are all guilty of spreading the episode further than we should. We are only human.

The only way out of the 'hole' is by getting excited about the little things in life. I found that pit the hard way by almost dying because I didn't want to be alive anymore. I thought they only way I was going to get out of being married was death. But I lived and started looking at writing as a career because it was natural for me.

Having a sense of humor is almost essential as a bipolar because if we took each even and looked at the negative effect it played on us, then the 'pity pot' always arrives. So, I made fun of my cell phone anxieties by mimicking what do in order to get proper signal at my residence, and I tell everyone that I had to plug the cell into the outside wall because the batter didn't last very long. As it was the winter season. I had to wear my parka, winter boots and gloves while waving the antenna with my right arm, holding my cell with my left asking, "Can you hear me now?" People laugh because they understand. I have to make fun of the dog because, it, to me is truly annoying with its Emmy award-winning pitiful look. My face transforms into what the dog looks like, and I get on all fours and act like I'm going to be beaten when I enter the residence. I also portray the dog as if it's talking to another 'guest' dog on the property and say "Thank God you're here! That evil woman made me sit in a corner the whole time you were gone! Please don't leave me behind again!" This too, the humor factor, allows people to laugh because they understand.

Having someone who understands you is like having another half- a person who relates to what you're going through. My support person is my adopted sister. She wasn't adopted into my birth family; I adopted her and her family as my own because they unconditionally love me just like unconditionally love them. It doesn't mean I wear rose colored glasses when it comes to my support family. I call them on their bad behaviours and my sister laughs at me when I talk animatedly about events that bug me. The great thing about having my sister is that we have an agreement; whining isn't really whining, it's venting, and there are no suggestions for improvement. Every person needs to vent. Life can be so overwhelming that venting is an absolute must.

When you have someone who says, 'I hear you and I can only imagine what you are going through. That must have sucked the big hairy hamster. Holy doodle! That sound rough." It helps so much, even if they don't have complete understanding of why the bipolar is so upset about something so minor. But empathy is the key to settling a bipolar down.

Picking a bipolar up and out of the hole is like giving shock therapy to a dying man. We need it, and I don't care what other bipolar say. When I'm down, having my sister say, "What the heck are you doing? Let's get back on the train and find a way. You have it in you now so stop whining and let's go already!" She also says, "Just kidding!" a lot. We balance each other out; we are like the proverbial yin and yang. When I'm up and excitable, she down, and vice versa. She makes sure I eat and care about me and for that alone I wouldn't give her up for the world. I don't care about the flaws she has. I have flaws and that doesn't make her love me less. If only the rest of the world was like mad sister and I, it would be a much better place.

You Can Never Have Too Much

Recognition
by Terri Kovalcik

let us not quibble over small
differences
let us rejoice
in our similarities
our friendship is quite nice

Information that is! There is quite a bit of information out there and support groups for the bipolar disordered. The more you know the better off you are, so with that in mind these are the websites that I went to and obtained factual information:

www.heretohelpbc.ca Fact Sheets – Bipolar Disorder

www.about.com Bipolar Disorder: Why So Many Classifications of Bipolar Disorder?

What is Bipolar 1 Disorder?

What is the Difference Between Bipolar 1 and 2 Disorder?

I'm Bipolar: Creativity Returns-But Socialbity Gone (7/18/99)

Eight Weeks After Diagnosis

Toxic People- How to Avoid Toxic People

Thoughtless or tactless things said about bipolar disorder can hurt

Top humorous gifts for Manci Depressive (you have to go here they have hilarious gifts)

How to Explain Bipolar Disorder to Others

Explaining Bipolar Disorder

Regaining Perspective; Bipolars and Loved Ones, Marriage & Manic Depression: Making it Work

ww.wtheonion.com God Diagnosed with Bipolar Disorder

www.pyschoeducation.ord. Depression, Bipolar 2 introduction

www.lollie.com How to be Depressed and How to be Happy

www.pendlum.org. Best Things to Say to Someone Who is Depressed

www.mentalhelath.com Bipolar Disorder.

www.nimh.nih.gov/publicat/index.cfm Bipolar Disorder with Addendum Bipolar January 2007 National Institute of Mental Health

There are other websites out there that I haven't discussed because there are far too many to name. One website I do encourage you to dead to, especially if you are financially able is bipolarcentral.com David Oliver, son of a bipolar mother, has written about how to repair relationships, finances, and other books that are helpful if you can afford them. I am hoping that one day I will be able to buy the books and CDs he has available.

The reality is that everything can be improved if everyone tries to make the choices that will enable this world to be a better place.

Understanding is the key!

www.ingramcontent.com/pod-product-compliance
Lightning Source LLC
Chambersburg PA
CBHW050523290526
45786CB00007B/2667